ATOPIC DERMATITIS

SOLVING ALL THE PUZZLES OF CURING

ATOPIC DERMATITIS

DR. J. SIMON

Contents

INTRODUCTION

Atopic dermatitis (AD), another name for eczema, is a chronic inflammatory skin illness characterized by itchy and inflamed skin. It usually appears on the skin as dry, red, and scaly patches. Although it is more common in children, atopic dermatitis is a widespread illness that can afflict people of any age. Although the precise cause of AD is unknown, immune system, environmental, and genetic factors are involved.

Vital Information About Atopic Dermatitis:

1. Warning signs:

Itching: Pruritus, or intense itching that may lead to scratching, is one of the primary signs and symptoms of atopic dermatitis.

Redness and Inflammation: Affected areas of the skin may flush, become inflamed, or even develop small lumps or blisters.

Dryness and Scaling: Skin with eczema frequently has a tendency to become dry, and it may also develop crusts or scales.

2. Typical Sites:

Often, atopic dermatitis affects the face, hands, elbows, and area behind the knees. It could affect a baby's cheeks and scalp.

3. Triggers:

The symptoms of AD can be brought on by or made worse by irritants (such as soaps or detergents), allergens (such as pollen or pet dander), stress, dry skin, and changes in humidity or temperature.

4. Date of Age Onset:

Atopic dermatitis can occur at any age, though it typically manifests in a child's early years. Many youngsters with AD either outgrow their condition or experience fewer symptoms as they get older.

5. Chronic Qualities:

Atopic dermatitis is a chronic condition that usually becomes worse with time. However, there could be periods when the symptoms go better and periods when they get worse.

6. Associated Conditions:

People with atopic dermatitis may also be more prone to other allergy problems such as asthma and hay fever, which contributes to the "atopic march."

7. Techniques of Care:

Medication, lifestyle modifications, and preventive measures are combined for management. Emollients, or moisturizers, topical corticosteroids, and systemic medications may be advised in severe cases.

8. Impact on the Quality of Life:

Atopic dermatitis can cause discomfort, emotional stress, and trouble sleeping, all of which can have a significant negative influence on quality of life. Social and everyday activities could also be affected.

9. Function of the immune system:

Both genetic predispositions and abnormal immune responses lead to atopic dermatitis. Dysregulation of the immune system leads to inflammation and breakdown of the skin barrier.

10. Present-day Studies:

The main objectives of ongoing study are to comprehend the fundamental causes of atopic dermatitis and develop customized therapies. Biologics and other advancements in treatment offer new hope for the care of severely ill individuals.

Effective care of atopic dermatitis requires a customized approach that takes into consideration the unique triggers and characteristics of each patient's condition. Although there is now no recognized treatment for atopic dermatitis, symptoms can be controlled and general health can be improved with the appropriate care and lifestyle changes.

CHAPTER ONE

Motives and Risk Factors

Multifactorial skin disease atopic dermatitis (AD) is influenced by immunological, environmental, and genetic factors. Acquiring understanding of the causes and contributing variables can aid in the development and management of AD. These are the primary factors associated with AD:

1. Biochemical Propensity:

Family history plays a significant role in the development of atopic dermatitis. Those with a family history of hay fever, allergic rhinitis, or asthma are more likely to suffer from the ailment. Numerous genetic variations related to immune response and skin barrier function affect susceptibility.

2. Immunological System Deficit:

Abnormal immune responses are one of the main causes of AD. Skin barrier breakdown and inflammation can occur when the immune system overreacts to environmental stimuli. Particularly Th2 cells, or T-helper cells, are implicated in the inflammatory processes connected to AD.

3. breakdown of the skin barrier

Skin barriers are usually compromised in people with atopic dermatitis, making the skin more vulnerable to allergens, irritants, and moisture loss. Proteins like filaggrin, which are crucial for maintaining the integrity of the skin, are deficient in, and skin barrier dysfunction is associated with these deficiencies.

4. Environmental Factors:

Allergens: Mold, dust mites, pollen, and pet dander are among the allergens that can aggravate or trigger symptoms of AD.

Irritants: Serums, fragrances, harsh detergents, and sturdy fabrics can irritate skin and lead to flare-ups.

Climate: Skin conditions can be brought on by changes in humidity, temperature, and exposure to extreme weather.

5. Microbiological Components:

Microbial dysbiosis: Modifications to the skin microbiome, such as an excess of certain bacteria, may contribute to the development or exacerbation of AD.

6. Early Life Exposures:

Early Antibiotic Use: Studies suggest that early exposure to antibiotics during infancy may be associated with an increased risk of AD.

Mode of Delivery: The beginning of AD may be influenced by the unique microorganisms that babies born via cesarean section may be exposed to.

7. Filaggrin mutations:

Mutations in the filaggrin gene, which is critical for maintaining the skin barrier, have been associated with a higher frequency of atopic dermatitis.

8. Psychological Components:

Stress: Two factors that may exacerbate AD symptoms are psychological and emotional stress. Stress-reduction strategies may be useful in the treatment of the condition.

9. Food allergies:

Food allergies and atopic dermatitis may be connected, albeit the relationship is not entirely evident. Understanding and managing specific food triggers may be crucial for a lot of people.

It's important to keep in mind that while these factors may increase the likelihood of atopic dermatitis, they do not guarantee that the condition will materialize. Additionally, the way that each person's unique blend of these traits interacts may vary. Avoiding triggers, following a skincare routine, and, in some cases, using medication to control symptoms are common ways to manage atopic dermatitis. Consultation with a dermatologist or other healthcare expert may help build a personalized management plan for AD based on specific circumstances.

Types and Subtypes

Atopic dermatitis (AD) can develop in various forms and subtypes, each with distinct characteristics and clinical presentations. Medical professionals can tailor treatment regimens to the specifics of each patient's AD thanks to the classification of the condition. The following are the main categories and subtypes of AD:

1. Childhood/Atopic Dermatitis in Infants:

Onset: Typically begins in the early years of life or infancy.

Location: Usually affects the face, scalp, and extensor surfaces (knees and elbows).

Features: Leaking and crusting red, itchy patches. Babies' cheeks and foreheads may display it.

2. Adult/teenage Atopic Dermatitis:

Origin: It might first show up in childhood and last into adolescence or adulthood, or it might start in childhood.

Location: Usually affects the hands, face, and neck, but it can also affect the flexural areas (behind the knees and inner elbows).

Characteristics: Periodic or recurring eczematous lesions that go through periods of remission.

3. dermatitis of the hands:

Location: Mostly the hands are affected.

Features: Red, scaly, dry patches on the hands that are itchy, unpleasant, and dry. Hand eczema may be brought on by irritants or allergens.

4. Discoid nummulous dermatitis:

Characteristics: Clearly defined, round (coin-shaped) lesions that could be scaly or crusty. often seen on the extremities.

5. Atheromatous eczema:

Characteristics: Often called "winter itch," it is characterized by dry, cracked skin, particularly in the elderly. often made worse by low humidity and chilly temps.

6. Contact dermatitis:

Features: Allergic contact dermatitis or irritant contact dermatitis is an inflammation of the skin brought on by contact with allergens or irritants. Coexisting dermatitis can occur between atopic and contact types.

7. Dermal thickening (Lichen Simplex Chronicus):

Features: Areas of the skin that have been repeatedly scraped or rubbed have hardened and turned leathery. usually noticed on the nape of the neck, wrists, or ankles.

8. Seborrheic dermatitis:

Features: Frequently affecting areas of the face and scalp with high sebaceous gland activity are red, scaly patches of irritation on the skin (dandruff).

9. dyshidrotic eczema:

Characteristics: Small, painful blisters on the hands and feet, often with redness and scaling. may be triggered by stress or certain medication exposure.

10. Stasis dermatitis:

Features: Eczema on the lower legs, typically associated with impaired circulation and persistent venous insufficiency. Possible symptoms include redness, swelling, and ulcerations.

It's important to keep in mind that people with atopic dermatitis may have a spectrum of symptoms and simultaneously display traits from multiple subtypes. Accurate diagnosis and categorization are essential for designing effective treatment plans that are tailored to the individual AD features and subtypes of each patient. A clear diagnosis and customized treatment plan should be obtained by consulting a dermatologist or other qualified healthcare provider.

Atopic dermatitis (AD) can have a wide range of intensity and dynamic signs and symptoms. The following traits are typical with AD:

1. Itching, or pruritus:

Severe itching is a common symptom of atopic dermatitis and is often the most bothersome aspect for the affected person.

2. Red or Inflamed Skin:

The affected areas of the skin could appear red, puffy, and sore. The redness is generally caused by an underlying inflammatory process.

3. Dry, scaly skin:

Patients with AD typically experience dry skin, which can occasionally turn scaly or develop rough, uneven patches.

4. Areas affected by eczema

The characteristic rash or patches associated with AD are referred to as "eczematous lesions". They could come in various sizes and shapes.

5. Crisp and Savvy:

During acute flare-ups, clear fluid may leak from the affected skin, and crusting may occur as the lesions dry.

6. Lichenification:

Repetitive scratching or rubbing can cause lichenification, a condition in which the skin becomes thicker, leathery, and hyperpigmented.

7. Together Participation:

AD commonly affects flexural regions, such as the space between the elbows and behind the knees. Certain areas may be more irritated, red, and itchy than others.

8. Participation of the Face:

In infants and children, atopic dermatitis commonly affects the face, particularly the cheeks and forehead. Adults may also experience symptoms in the eyes and neck.

9. Papules and Blisters:

During severe flare-ups, little raised lumps known as papules and blisters may develop. These could affect the overall texture of the skin.

10. Disturbances in sleep:

Itching and pain associated with AD can interfere with sleep, which can make patients weary and worsen the condition's consequences on daily living.

11. Allergy-ridden Shiners:

Allergy shiners, or dark circles or discoloration beneath the eyes, can be brought on by inflammation and rubbing of the eyes.

12. The Atopic Pleat in Dennie-Morgan Folding

The Dennie-Morgan fold, also known as the atopic pleat, is an extra fold or line that appears beneath the lower eyelid and may be a subtle indicator of atopic dermatitis.

It's important to keep in mind that symptoms of AD might vary from person to person and can change over time. Some of the factors that could lead to flare-ups include infections, stress, and exposure to irritants or allergens. Identifying triggers, establishing a consistent skincare routine, taking prescription medications (such as immunomodulators or topical corticosteroids), and attending to any underlying causes of the condition can all help treat atopic dermatitis. Anyone experiencing signs of AD should see a dermatologist or other healthcare provider for an accurate diagnosis and advice for a personalized treatment plan.

The primary methods for diagnosing atopic dermatitis (AD) include clinical examination, medical history, and occasionally further testing to rule out other skin conditions. Below is a summary of the AD diagnostic and evaluation process:

1. Background Information on Health:

A comprehensive medical history is necessary to comprehend the patient's symptoms, including when they began, how long they lasted, and any possible exacerbating or precipitating events. It's also critical to be aware of family history, allergies, and previous medical procedures.

2. Physical Evaluation:

A thorough physical examination of the skin is done to identify any lesions, their characteristics, and any regions of redness, scaling, or lichenification. The pattern and distribution of skin involvement are taken into consideration because AD often has a specific distribution.

3. Standards for Diagnosis:

The diagnosis of AD is often aided by recognized diagnostic criteria, such as the Hanifin and Rajka criteria or those established by the American Academy of Dermatology (AAD). These criteria consider whether specific symptoms exist, how they manifest, and their physical characteristics.

4. Not Included Are Any Other Conditions:

It's important to screen out other skin conditions that can present with similar symptoms. To rule out illnesses including psoriasis, seborrheic dermatitis, fungal infections, and contact dermatitis, clinical investigations should be performed.

5. Patch testing:

Patch testing is a useful tool for identifying potential allergens that may be contributing to AD symptoms. When allergic reactions or contact dermatitis are suspected, this is particularly crucial.

6. Laboratory Tests:

A patient may have a variety of laboratory tests to rule out other illnesses and assess their general health, even though there are no specific blood testing for AD. These could include complete blood count (CBC), erythrocyte sedimentation rate (ESR), and specific IgE testing for allergies.

7. Skin Biopsy: Rarely

In rare cases, a skin biopsy may be required to differentiate AD from other skin disorders. However, biopsies are typically not required for the conventional diagnosis of AD.

8. Assessment of Intensity:

Medical practitioners may assess the severity of AD in order to guide treatment decisions. This assessment considers factors such as the extent of skin involvement, the intensity of itching, the impact on daily activities, and the person's quality of life.

9. Following and Observation:

Regular monitoring and follow-up appointments are necessary to assess the response to treatment, adjust the management plan, and address any emerging problems. When employing this collaborative technique, there needs to be ongoing contact between the patient and the healthcare provider.

To develop an effective AD treatment plan, a precise diagnosis and evaluation are necessary. Dermatologists, allergists, and other medical specialists that specialize in treating skin disorders are primarily responsible for the diagnosis and treatment of atopic dermatitis. People experiencing symptoms suggestive of AD should seek professional examination for a correct diagnosis and customized therapy.

Things that aggravate and set off

There are numerous triggers and aggravating events that can exacerbate Atopic Dermatitis (AD) symptoms and lead to flare-ups. It is necessary to comprehend these triggers and learn how to control them in order to effectively manage AD.

CHAPTER TWO

The following are common circumstances and factors that exacerbate AD:

1. Allergens:

Exposure to allergens can cause or worsen symptoms of AD. Common allergies include:

- Pollen
- Pet dander
- dust mites
- mold

2. irritants:

Skin sensitivity from irritating substances can exacerbate AD. Common irritants include:

- strong soaps and detergents
- perfumed products
- Wool or synthetic fabrics
- chemicals present in cleaning supplies

3. Type of Dry Skin:

Dry skin is a common cause for AD. Maintaining moisturized skin is crucial to preventing flare-ups.

4. Weather Update:

Variations in the weather, particularly low humidity and cold temperatures, can make AD symptoms worse and result in dry skin. Hot weather and excessive perspiration may also make symptoms worse.

5. Emphasize

Emotional stress might be a major trigger for AD flare-ups. Stress management techniques may mitigate its damaging impact on the skin.

6. infections

Skin infections, particularly those brought on by bacteria or viruses, might aggravate AD symptoms or cause them to worsen. It's critical to treat infections as quickly as possible.

7. alterations in hormones

Hormonal changes, such as those that occur during puberty or pregnancy, can have an impact on AD symptoms.

8. Foods:

Some persons with AD may be provoked by certain foods, though this is less common. Common food triggers include:

- dairy products
- Eggs
- Nuts
- Shellfish
- Wheat

9. Clothing:

Certain materials and form-fitting clothing can irritate the skin. Selecting materials that are pliable and flexible can be beneficial.

10. Itching

Scratching the affected skin region may make the condition worse and result in lichenification, or thickening of the skin.

11. Being overheated:

Prolonged heat exposure or overheating can cause sweating, which exacerbates discomfort and irritation.

12. Responses Intolerant to:

Exposure to chemicals that trigger allergic reactions may result in AD symptoms. This category may include allergens found in personal hygiene products, scents, and cosmetics.

13. Disturbances in sleep:

An erratic sleep schedule or poor quality of sleep can be the cause of AD flare-ups.

14. Smoking:

Tobacco smoke may exacerbate AD symptoms. The best course of action is to avoid smoking and secondhand smoke.

It can be essential to keep an extensive log of symptoms and potential exposures in order to identify each person's particular triggers. Effective symptom management and exposure reduction techniques can be put into place after triggers have been identified. Good skincare, avoiding triggers, and, in some cases, medication are all part of a complex strategy that is commonly used to treat AD and improve the overall quality of life for persons who have this condition. Consulting with a dermatologist or other healthcare expert can assist tailor a management plan according to particular needs.

Techniques for Counseling

To effectively treat Atopic Dermatitis (AD), a comprehensive approach that addresses both acute flare-ups and long-term symptom control is required. When developing treatment plans, considerations include the patient's response to certain interventions, the degree of symptoms, and individual triggers. The following are crucial components of treatment strategies for AD:

1. Skincare and Hydration:

Emollients: Regular application of emollients, such as moisturizers and ointments, helps to maintain the skin's moisture content and fortifies its outermost layer. After a bath, emollients are most effective when applied immediately.

2. Applying Corticosteroids Locally:

Anti-Inflammatory Creams: Topical corticosteroids are often used to alleviate inflammation during acute flare-ups. Based on the severity of symptoms, the dosage and length of usage should be determined. Additionally, they should be used under a healthcare provider's supervision.

3. Topical Calcineurin Inhibitors:

Immunomodulators: Topical calcineurin inhibitors, such as tacrolimus and pimecrolimus, are safe alternatives to anti-inflammatory medications for use on the face and other sensitive areas of the body.

4. Pharmaceuticals for the System:

Oral Antihistamines: Non-sedating antihistamines may be recommended to assist reduce itching and improve sleep.

Oral Corticosteroids: In severe situations, a short-term prescription for oral corticosteroids may be given to treat acute flare-ups. However, extended use is typically discouraged due to potential negative effects.

5. Wet Wrap Therapy:

Moisturizing and Calming Wraps: As part of wet wrap therapy, emollients and moisturizing bandages are applied to affected regions, helping to hydrate the skin and reduce inflammation. This is often done under medical supervision.

6. Phototherapy or light therapy:

UVB or UVA Light Exposure: Under medical supervision, regulated exposure to UVB or UVA light may be beneficial in the treatment of moderate-to-severe AD.

7. Dupilumab, a biologic medication:

IL-4 Receptor Antagonist: Dupilumab, a biologic medication, inhibits the actions of some immune system components associated with AD. It is typically used when all other therapeutic options have failed.

8. Identifying and Managing Stressors

Avoiding allergies: By identifying and avoiding specific allergies or triggers, such as certain foods or environmental situations, you can help prevent flare-ups.

9. Behavioral Techniques:

Stress management techniques, such as mindfulness, meditation, and stress reduction, may be beneficial in managing AD, as stress is a known trigger for the illness.

10. Immunotherapy Based on Antigens:

Allergy injections (desensitization): When specific allergens have been identified, allergen immunotherapy may be taken into consideration in order to desensitize the immune system.

11. Intervention with Antimicrobials:

Antibiotics or Antivirals: In cases when bacterial or viral infections are present, antimicrobial therapy may be advised.

12. Avoid Bringing Up Irritants:

Irritant Avoidance: You can prevent the worsening of your symptoms by limiting your exposure to irritants, such as soaps and strong detergents.

The AD treatment regimen for each patient is unique and tailored to their needs. Setting up regular follow-up appointments with doctors is essential for determining the effectiveness of treatments, adjusting medications as needed, and dealing with any emerging problems. Making lifestyle adjustments such as avoiding triggers and adhering to a regular skincare routine are critical to the overall management of AD. Patients are advised to engage in active communication with their healthcare team to ensure that the treatment plan suits their requirements and preferences.

Considerations for Lifestyle and Skincare

Atopic Dermatitis (AD) management requires both lifestyle changes and proper skincare regimens. These techniques aim to lessen stress, moisturize the skin, and improve overall health. Important skincare and lifestyle considerations for those with AD include the following:

1. Apply moisturizer frequently:

Apply emollients, ointments, and moisturizers multiple times a day, especially after bathing. Select fragrance-free goods with minimal ingredient lists to avoid potential sensitivities.

2. Simple Cleaning:

Instead of using strong detergents or soaps, utilize mild cleansers without any scent. For your bath or shower, use warm water and set a timer. Pat the skin dry as opposed to rubbing it with a cloth.

3. Choose Apprising Apparel:

Choose airy, loose-fitting clothes composed of cotton or other soft materials. Steer clear of wool and synthetic fabrics that could irritate your skin.

4. Steer clear of triggers:

Determine and stay away from particular triggers, such as allergies, harsh chemicals, or particular materials, that exacerbate the symptoms of AD. This can entail staying away from known allergies and washing clothes with hypoallergenic detergents.

5. Manage Your Tension:

Use stress-reduction strategies including yoga, meditation, and deep breathing. Reducing stress can enhance general wellbeing and aid in the prevention of flare-ups.

6. Keep Your Skincare Routine Uniform:

Create a regular skincare regimen that includes moisturizing and any necessary medicines. To properly manage AD, consistency is essential.

7. Control of Humidity and Temperature:

Keep the inside climate cozy by keeping the humidity and temperature under control. Low humidity and extreme temperatures can worsen the symptoms of dry skin.

8. Control of Allergens:

Use strategies to limit your exposure to common allergens, like cleaning your home on a regular basis and using bedding covers that are allergen-proof.

9. Sun Protection:

For skin protection against sun exposure, use sunscreen with a high SPF. AD flare-ups can be triggered by sunburn. Select a sunscreen that is appropriate for skin that is sensitive.

10. Steer clear of scratching:

Cut short nails to reduce the risk of skin abrasions from rubbing. To stop youngsters from scratching too much as they sleep, try using gloves or anti-scratch mittens for babies.

11. Wet Wrap Therapy:

Wet wrap therapy can be used as a targeted treatment for severe flare-ups under medical supervision. To soothe the skin, it entails applying moist bandages and emollients to the afflicted areas.

12. Steer clear of allergens:

If testing reveals a particular allergy, reduce exposure to it through food and/or environmental factors.

13. Frequent Examinations:

Make routine follow-up meetings with a dermatologist or other healthcare professional to discuss any concerns, monitor the condition, and modify treatment strategies.

14. Conducting Allergy Testing:

Take into account allergy testing to find possible causes. Strategies for avoiding allergens can be guided by this information.

15. Assisted by Healthcare Providers:

Work together with medical professionals to address new problems, customize the treatment plan to each patient's needs, and investigate novel therapeutic approaches.

The overall management of AD requires careful consideration of these skincare and lifestyle factors. For those with AD, minimizing flare-ups, increasing treatment efficacy, and improving overall quality of life are all possible with a proactive and consistent approach. It is crucial to seek the advice of medical professionals for tailored advice depending on specific situations.

Coping strategies and emotional well-being

In addition to treating the physical symptoms of Atopic Dermatitis (AD), coping with the condition also entails addressing its emotional effects. Having a chronic skin condition can have an impact on one's emotional health, body image, and self-worth. The following coping mechanisms arc intended to improve the emotional resilience and general well-being of people with AD:

1. Understanding and knowledge:

Learn everything there is to know about AD, including its causes and prevention techniques. Acquiring knowledge enables people to actively participate in their own care.

2. Providing a Network of Support:

Create a network of friends, family, and medical professionals who can support you. Talk to others that can empathize and provide support about your struggles, victories, and experiences.

3. Support Teams:

Participate in online or in-person AD support groups to meet people going through similar struggles. It can be reassuring and empowering to share coping mechanisms and experiences.

4. Honest Communication

Openly discuss your physical and mental wellness with your medical professionals. Talk about how AD affects relationships, daily living, and mental health.

5. Techniques for Stress Management:

Engage in stress-relieving exercises like yoga, mindfulness, meditation, and deep breathing. Controlling stress can enhance general quality of life and help avoid flare-ups.

6. Good Lifestyle Decisions:

Embrace a healthy lifestyle that includes enough sleep, a balanced diet, and frequent exercise.

These elements support general health and have a beneficial effect on AD symptoms.

7. Psychoanalysis and Counseling:

In order to deal with the emotional effects of AD, think about getting help from a therapist or counselor. Tools for managing stress, worry, and the difficulties of having a chronic illness can be obtained through therapy.

8. Self-Helding:

Make enjoyable and calming self-care activities a priority. This can involve things like reading, having a bath, engaging in a pastime, or going outside.

9. Gratitude and Awareness:

Take up mindfulness exercises and work on accepting your circumstance. Instead of wallowing in regrets for the past or anxieties for the future, concentrate on the here and now.

10. Set logical goals:

Establish attainable targets for managing AD. Appreciate little accomplishments and advancements, and practice self-compassion when facing difficult days.

11. Body-Aware Mentality:

Develop a positive sense of self-worth and body image. Realize that self-worth and beauty go beyond outward appearances.

12. Expert Assistance:

Seek advice from experts when necessary, including dermatologists, allergists, and mental health specialists. Taking a multidisciplinary approach can help address AD's emotional and physical components.

13. Writing a Journal:

Write in a journal to document symptoms, process feelings, and consider everyday events. This can be used as a tool for introspection and dialogue with medical professionals.

14. Accomplishments with honor:

Celebrate and acknowledge individual accomplishments, whether they are in the form of reaching goals, conquering obstacles, or effectively managing symptoms.

15. Creative Recess:

Take up creative pursuits or hobbies as a way to express yourself and let go of your emotions. This could apply to writing, music, or art.

The road of coping with AD is comprehensive, involving both mental and physical health. Through the integration of these coping methods, as well as obtaining assistance from medical professionals and a community that supports them, people with AD can improve their resilience and lead satisfying lives.

Youngsters and AD

Atopic Dermatitis (AD) is a prevalent cutaneous ailment that frequently commences during childhood. In order to effectively manage AD in children, parents, caregivers, and medical professionals must work together. For kids with AD, keep the following in mind:

1. Early Detection

Red, itchy spots on the face, scalp, and extensor surfaces are common early signs of AD in infants. Effective management requires early detection and intervention.

2. Skincare regimen:

Provide the youngster with a gentle and consistent skincare regimen. To keep your skin hydrated, use hypoallergenic and fragrance-free products and moisturize frequently.

3. Steer clear of triggers:

Recognize and stay away from possible triggers, such as allergies, strong detergents, and particular textiles. As much as you can, keep the child's surroundings free of allergens.

4. Options for Clothes:

To reduce irritation, wear loose-fitting, breathable, and soft clothing made of natural materials like cotton.

5. Testing for Allergens:

To determine which specific allergens may be causing flare-ups, think about being tested for allergies. Strategies for avoiding allergens can be guided by this information.

6. Use of Emollients:

After taking a bath, apply emollients right away to seal in moisture. Emollients prevent dryness and soothe the skin.

7. Bathing Methods:

To prevent drying out the skin, take baths in lukewarm water and don't spend too much time in the tub. Pat dry the child's skin rather than dabbing at it with a towel.

8. Pediatric-Friendly Drugs:

It is important to apply topical corticosteroids and other prescribed medications according to the doctor's instructions. Select kid-friendly formulas and talk to the provider about any worries you may have.

9. Wet Wrap Therapy:

When used under medical supervision, wet wrap therapy can be a successful intervention for children experiencing severe flare-ups. Emollients and moist bandages are applied to the affected areas.

10. Handling Itches:

Teach kids age-appropriate methods to control their itching, like using a cold compress or distraction tactics. Cut short nails to reduce the chance of skin irritation from rubbing.

11. Sun Protection:

To shield the child's skin from the sun, apply sunscreen with a high SPF. Select a sunscreen that is safe for delicate skin.

12. Bedrooms Free of Allergens:

Use hypoallergenic bedding covers and routinely clean the bedroom to create a sleeping environment free of allergens.

13. Encouragement in the School Environment:

Talk about the child's condition with the staff and teachers at the school. Ascertain that the school environment is encouraging and that appropriate skincare is practiced during the day.

14. Psychological Support:

Offer the child emotional support, attending to any issues with body image, social interactions, or self-esteem. Promote honest dialogue.

15. Dermatologist for children:

See a pediatric dermatologist if you need specialized treatment. Pediatric dermatologists are skilled in treating children's skin conditions.

It's critical that parents and other caregivers collaborate closely with medical professionals to create a customized management plan for every child with AD. A comprehensive approach to managing childhood AD includes regular follow-up appointments, making modifications to the treatment plan, and addressing any emotional concerns.

Pregnancy and Family Planning

Those with atopic dermatitis (AD) who are expecting or intend to start a family may need to take special considerations. Taking into account the possible effects on the mother and the unborn child as well as the available treatment options is crucial when managing AD during pregnancy. The following are crucial factors to take into account when planning a family and getting pregnant in AD:

1. Talking with the healthcare provider:

It's important to speak with your healthcare provider if you have AD and intend to get pregnant or if you are already pregnant. They are able to offer tailored advice according to your particular circumstances.

2. Examining the medication:

Talk to your healthcare provider about the medications you currently take. During pregnancy, certain commonly prescribed medications for AD management, like calcineurin inhibitors and topical corticosteroids, may need to be changed or substituted with safer options.

3. Skincare Items Safe During Pregnancy:

Choose skincare products safe for pregnancy that don't contain any potentially dangerous ingredients. Emollients and moisturizers can be used to treat dry skin brought on by AD.

4. Stress Non-Pharmacological Methods:

Prioritize non-pharmacological methods to reduce the need for prescription drugs during pregnancy, such as good skincare, avoiding triggers, and stress management.

5. Testing for Allergens:

To pinpoint particular triggers and enable targeted avoidance tactics during pregnancy, think about conducting allergen testing.

6. Sun Protection:

Pregnancy-safe sunscreen should be used to protect against the sun. Sun protection is crucial because exposure to the sun may exacerbate the symptoms of AD.

7. Hormonal Changes Associated with Pregnancy:

Recognize that AD symptoms may be impacted by hormonal changes associated with pregnancy.

While some people might see an improvement, others might experience an aggravation. It's crucial to closely monitor with a healthcare professional.

8. Handling Itches:

Use itch-management techniques, like cold compresses, to ease pregnancy discomforts.

9. Support for Mental Health:

In addition to the emotional strain that comes with being pregnant, managing a chronic illness like AD can be stressful. If you require mental health support, get it, and be honest with your medical team about any emotional issues you may be having.

10. Things to Think About When Breastfeeding:

If you are nursing, find out from your doctor if any topical treatments for AD are safe to take while nursing. Topical treatments are generally regarded as safe, though specific situations may differ.

11. Organizing Prior to Fertility:

Talk to your healthcare provider about preconception planning if family planning is being considered. Pregnancy health can be enhanced by maintaining optimum health prior to conception.

12. Consultation with Pediatric Dermatologists:

When considering starting a family, take into account speaking with a pediatric dermatologist if AD runs in the family. They can address any worries about a genetic predisposition and offer advice on how to manage AD in children.

13. A Home Free of Allergens:

Establish a home free of allergens to lessen possible triggers both before and after the baby is born.

14. Itch Relief Safe for Pregnancy:

Examine methods of relieving itching that are safe to use during pregnancy, such as taking cool baths, dressing loosely, and using a humidifier to avoid dry air.

15. Frequent Examinations:

Make time for routine check-ups with your healthcare provider to ensure the health and wellbeing of the unborn child throughout your pregnancy.

The secret is to collaborate closely with your medical team to create a thorough and unique plan that puts the mother's and the baby's health first. For those with AD, a successful and healthy pregnancy is facilitated by open communication, routine check-ups, and management plan modifications as necessary.

CHAPTER FOUR

While medical professionals' prescribed conventional treatments are crucial in the management of Atopic Dermatitis (AD), some people choose to investigate complementary complementary therapies and home remedies. It is crucial to remember that in order to make sure alternative therapies are safe and work well with the entire treatment plan, they should be discussed with healthcare providers. The following are some alternative and DIY treatments that people with AD might want to think about:

1. Probiotics:

Beneficial bacteria called probiotics may help to maintain gut health. There may be a connection between gut health and AD, according to some studies. Consult a medical professional before starting a probiotic regimen.

2. Coconut Oil:

Moisturizing the skin can be achieved by applying virgin coconut oil to the affected areas. It might possess antibacterial and anti-inflammatory qualities. It is advised to perform patch testing to guarantee compatibility.

3. Oil of Evening Primrose:

Some people think that evening primrose oil, which is high in gamma-linolenic acid (GLA), has anti-inflammatory qualities. Be sure to speak with a doctor before taking it as a supplement.

4. Baths with oatmeal:

Baths with colloidal oatmeal can relieve itching and calm irritated skin. After taking a bath, make sure the water is lukewarm and pat the skin dry.

5. Dear Honey:

Applying manuka honey topically can help soothe skin because of its potential antibacterial and anti-inflammatory properties. But proceed with caution and seek medical advice, particularly if the person has allergies.

6. Aloe vera

Straight from the plant, aloe vera gel can be applied to soothe irritated skin and may have a cooling effect. Inspect for allergies and confer with a medical professional.

7. Baths with bleach:

Diluted bleach baths are suggested by certain medical professionals as a possible way to lessen bacterial colonization on the skin. Only someone with medical supervision should perform this.

8. acupuncture

In acupuncture, tiny needles are inserted into predetermined body points in accordance with traditional Chinese medical protocol. Some people find it useful for stress management, which has an effect on the symptoms of AD.

9. The use of hypnosis

Hypnotherapy could be investigated as an additional strategy to reduce stress and enhance general wellbeing. Speak with a trained professional.

10. Mindfulness and Meditation:

Relaxation methods and mindfulness meditation can help control stress, which may lessen its negative effects on AD symptoms.

11. Dietary Adjustments:

Some people look into making dietary adjustments, like cutting out foods that might trigger an attack or adding foods that reduce inflammation. For individualized advice, speak with a registered dietitian or healthcare professional.

12. Supplementing with Vitamin D:

Sufficient levels of vitamin D are critical for healthy skin. Consult a medical professional to determine whether vitamin D supplementation is necessary.

13. Cream of calendula:

The cream called calendula, which is made from marigold flowers, is thought to have anti-inflammatory qualities. It is advisable to talk with a healthcare provider about the use of patch testing.

14. Meditation and Yoga:

Mind-body exercises like yoga and meditation can help lower stress and improve general wellbeing. To guarantee safety, speak with a healthcare professional.

15. Essential Oils:

Some essential oils, such as lavender or chamomile, are believed to have calming properties. To avoid irritating the skin, they should be used sparingly and diluted as needed. Consult with a healthcare provider before using essential oils.

It's crucial to approach alternative therapies with caution and seek guidance from healthcare providers. What works for one person may not work for another, and individual responses to alternative treatments can vary. It's recommended to discuss any alternative therapies or home remedies with a healthcare provider to ensure they are safe, appropriate, and compatible with the overall management of AD.

CONCLUSION

In conclusion, Atopic Dermatitis (AD) is a chronic inflammatory skin condition that requires a comprehensive and individualized approach to management. Key factors of controlling AD include:

Skincare regimen:

Establishing a consistent and mild skincare routine, including the use of emollients and moisturizers, is vital for maintaining skin hydrated and preventing flare-ups.

Medical Treatments:

Topical corticosteroids, calcineurin inhibitors, and other recommended drugs play a major role in treating inflammation and symptoms. Systemic medicines, phototherapy, and biologic therapies may be tried in extreme situations.

Identification and Avoidance of Triggers:

Identifying and avoiding triggers, such as allergies, irritants, and stress, is vital for reducing exacerbations of AD.

Lifestyle Considerations:

Adopting a healthy lifestyle, including regular exercise, a balanced diet, and stress management, adds to general well-being and may positively improve AD symptoms.

Childbearing and Family Organization:

Individuals with AD who are pregnant or planning a family should work closely with healthcare practitioners to develop a safe and effective management plan that emphasizes the well-being of both the mother and the baby.

Alternative Therapies and Home Remedies:

While alternative therapies and home remedies may be investigated as complimentary options, it's crucial to discuss these with healthcare experts to verify they are safe and compatible with the overall treatment plan.

Emotional Well-Being:

Coping methods, mental health support, and open communication with healthcare providers contribute to emotional well-being in individuals with AD.

Pediatric Considerations:

Managing AD in children entails early detection, a mild skincare routine, and collaboration with healthcare specialists to guarantee optimal treatment during childhood.

Ongoing Follow-Up:

Regular follow-up consultations with healthcare experts are necessary for monitoring symptoms, changing treatment programs, and addressing any emergent issues.

Holistic Approach:

A holistic strategy that incorporates both the physical and emotional components of AD is vital for attaining long-term management and increasing the quality of life for those with this condition.

It's crucial for individuals with AD to work together with dermatologists, allergists, and other healthcare specialists to develop a complete management strategy that suits their unique needs. By staying informed, adopting good lifestyle behaviors, and obtaining timely medical assistance, individuals with AD can effectively manage the condition and have satisfying lives.

THE END

www.ingramcontent.com/pod-product-compliance
Lightning Source LLC
Chambersburg PA
CBHW050743260726
48661CB00001B/388